# Healthy and fit with autophagy

*How to boost your health, lose body fat, prevent disease and look younger with autophagy*

Sebastian Thiele

# CONTENTS

# What you can expect in this book

What do you think of when you hear the word recycling? No doubt you immediately think of a few things to do with nature conservation, the reuse of non-degradable raw materials or waste and waste recycling. You might want to stop reading here because you don't want to be lectured on climate protection and sustainability any more than you already are in the media. But did you know that our bodies also have millions of small "recycling points"? Sure, the whole thing sounds very implausible at first, but the further you read in this book - and it really is worth it - the more impressed you will be and the clearer it will become to you what a masterpiece our body is and how much you can still learn from it and about it.

As you readers are probably not all at the same level of knowledge, you can read more about the body's own metabolic process in the cells and the biological background on the first few pages of the book, before moving on to the actual topic - the recycling process of cells, also known as autophagy. But so that you don't put the book back straight away because you had already had enough of cells at school and didn't understand a thing, here is the all-clear:

You don't have to be afraid of complicated chemical and biological processes or complicated technical language with incredibly convoluted sentences. Wisely anticipating that these small cells, which in an incredible way determine your whole life, are not so easy to understand, the book slowly and gradually leads you further and further into the subject and, following a theoretical part that is easy to understand even for laypeople, you can learn even more about the practical benefits of autophagy in medicine and even take action yourself and do something for your own health. So what are you waiting for? Get started and learn how you can already do something about dementia, cancer and old age.

# The cell - the smallest common multiple

## A BRIEF PROFILE

Before things really get going, you may be asking yourself what exactly a cell is. You may even remember your biology lessons from school and the oft-repeated mnemonic "Mitochondria are the power plants of cells". But that's where it gets difficult. Cell nucleus, endoplasmic reticulum, Golgi apparatus and much more probably didn't even occur to you spontaneously, although without all these small components you wouldn't be able to hold this book in your hand, read it, let alone live. To refresh your memory a little and perhaps add one or two things, you will find a few more explanations on the following pages. But so that it doesn't get too complex right at the beginning, you can also compare the cell to a large factory and thus perhaps better visualize how and what happens in the cell.

In a cell, there are many individual cell organelles, each of which has a different task. In your factory, the organelles would correspond to individual departments, all of which work to ensure that the factory functions as a whole. The most important cell organelle is the **cell nucleus**, where DNA is stored and copied. These copies are then either converted into amino acids and proteins to create cell organelles or information, and remain within the cell, or are used for cell duplication. For your factory, the cell nucleus would be like the **boss's office**, which has the instructions for all the work steps and the important information for the individual departments. He can now either copy some of these instructions and information in order to distribute them to the workstations within the factory, or he can use the entire copy to build a new second factory. As you can see, without a cell nucleus, nothing works in the cell, because if the instructions for all the basic steps are missing, no work can be done.

The aforementioned "power plants of the cells", the **mitochondria,** are also very important for the cell. These provide the cell with enough energy to perform all its tasks successfully. In your factory, the mitochondria might be the snacks and packed lunches for the employees or the energy for machines in the form of electricity.

The **endoplasmic reticulum**, which forms proteins and passes them on to the **Golgi apparatus so that** they can either be released from the cell or incorporated into the cell itself, also becomes important in the course of the process. The two organelles together are therefore almost like a small post station that either passes on products developed in the factory to other factories that need the products or distributes the products in its own factory to support departments or carry out further work steps.

When talking about autophagy, however, you must not forget the **lysosomes**, which break down unnecessary substances so that the resulting raw materials can then be reused. However, the lysosomes can not only break down the cell's own substances, but also absorb substances from the environment and "recycle" them or, in the case of toxic substances or attackers such as bacteria or viruses, destroy them and break them down into their individual parts. In your factory, a system like this would certainly also be an advantage, as you would not have to buy everything new, you could save raw materials and money and even protect your factory from attackers and hackers.

To summarize once again, remember that the cell nucleus provides the information, the mitochondria provide the energy, the endoplasmic reticulum and the Golgi apparatus together serve as the mail and distribute products and information from the cell nucleus within the cell or to the outside, and the lysosomes are the "eco-freaks" who do not want to throw away any raw material without first checking that it is really no longer usable. All organelles are closely connected to each other and as soon as one part no longer functions and cannot be repaired, the whole cell is destroyed.

But wait, before you read on, you need to know about a very important part of the cells that forms the basis for all metabolic processes, because without a **cell wall** that shields the cell from its environment, none of this would be possible. In your factory, you also need a few walls, doors and windows so that not just anyone can come into the factory and take what they need. You also need to protect your factory from environmental influences such as rain, snow, heat or even a storm or flood. And you certainly don't want your products to simply spread uncontrollably throughout the area and end up with nothing left. The same applies to the cells, because they don't want anything to be stolen from them, to be damaged by environmental conditions or for the laboriously produced cell products to be distributed without having a function. Each cell has therefore developed a small wall that protects it from all these things. If the cell region is flooded with nutrients, for example, the cell can protect itself from this and decide for itself via channels in its wall how much it wants to let through or not. This also applies to transport out of the cell, as cells can also produce things that they do not need themselves, but are only needed in other areas. If the cell then wants to release something to the outside, it can open its channels and export the desired substances.

You can imagine it all as a huge organism that is divided into many small units. If the organism provides substances, each unit can decide for itself whether it needs this substance or not. And if the organism notices that something is missing in one part of it, it can even make other parts aware of this and ask the units to support each other. Isn't it incredible how much these little cells can do? Wouldn't that be an example

that the global economy could take a leaf out of its
book?

# THE DHL OF CELLS

Now that you have already learned a lot about cells and have refreshed your knowledge a little, you can delve deeper into the topic and look at metabolism and transport in the cell. As you can perhaps imagine, the cell cannot produce all the products it needs itself, but must also absorb things from the environment and incorporate them into the cell. After all, a factory cannot function without a constant exchange with the environment in the form of imports and exports. New raw materials are constantly being delivered and finished products shipped. And this is exactly how it works in the cell. There are many different types of transportation, which you can take a closer look at below.

First of all, the uptake into the cell, **endocytosis,** which can be further subdivided into pinocytosis and phagocytosis. These terms probably sound very complex to you at first and you are wondering how you are supposed to understand all this. But don't worry, the whole thing is simpler than it sounds and you only need a brief overview of the individual types of transport. The difference between the two types of uptake really only lies in the type of substance that is absorbed. Pinocytosis involves soluble products and phagocytosis involves whole particles, bacteria, foreign bodies and similar larger items. As a little mnemonic, you can also remember that pinocytosis is the shorter word and therefore smaller products are ingested. Phagocytosis, on the other hand, is the longer word and larger particles are ingested as a whole. And endocytosis in general always means that something is transported into the cells.

Another transport option is **transcytosis,** which only transports substances through a cell without releasing them to the respective cell. The substance is therefore taken up on one side and released on the opposite side. At this moment, you can compare the cell to a small obstacle and since it would be more complicated and perhaps impossible to bypass this obstacle due to neighboring cells, the substance is simply passed through. Isn't it amazing what the cell can do?

The last important transport is **exocytosis**, through which substances that have been produced in the cell and are needed elsewhere in the body are excreted. In your company, this would be the export of finished products or products that are further processed in other factories.

So you can see that cell transport can be differentiated between endocytosis, transcytosis and exocytosis, whereby endocytosis can also be subdivided into pinocytosis and phagocytosis. So it's not as complicated as it seems at first glance. But what does all this transportation have to do with the many recycling yards you heard about earlier? You can find the answer to this legitimate question in the next few very interesting and surprising chapters.

# Recycling in Mini

## THE QUEST FOR INDEPENDENCE

As a child and now as an adult, you probably often thought that you wanted to do all your tasks on your own and ideally do everything perfectly and without help. You wanted to be independent and prove to those around you that you were strong enough to take on all the hurdles on your own. And to be honest, there are many advantages to mastering things on your own and not being dependent on others and help. And it is precisely this independence that your cells strive for. Dependence on others makes the cells vulnerable and unstable, because as soon as an important source is lost, the whole organism no longer functions. What's more, just like in your factory, all this transportation that you learned so much about earlier does not happen without losses. Not only can loads be damaged during transportation, it is also time-consuming and costs raw materials and energy. The products have to be packaged accordingly, they have to be transported and wouldn't it be much nicer if everything could take place in the cell and the cells were independent - just as you wanted?

And this is exactly what nature has taken care of and fulfilled the cells' wish by giving each cell its own recycling system so that it can reuse products that are no longer needed, thus creating a cycle in which other cells and their products play no role at all.

# AUTOPHAGY - SELF-DECOMPOSI-
TION

The Japanese scientist Yoshinori Ōsumi was even a-warded a Nobel Prize for his discovery of the process of autophagy, which, translated as self-decomposition, sounds very daunting. When he began his research in the early 1990s, only a few scientists were working on this topic, so Yoshinori Ōsumi had free rein to discover everything you are about to find out in the next few minutes.

Hidden behind the difficult-to-understand term autophagy is an intracellular process by which the cell's own products, which are either defective or no longer needed, are broken down. This enables the cell to make optimum use of all resources and not waste anything, because the cells cannot afford to do so. In a highly complex process, these waste products are packaged into so-called autophagosomes, which then fuse with lysosomes and become autolysosomes.

But before this goes too far into depth, the most important point to remember is that autolysosomes keep the breakdown of old cell products and the production of new ones in balance. This allows the cells to rejuvenate themselves again and again by simply breaking down old and worn-out components into their individual parts and then reassembling them. Wouldn't it be good if humans were also capable of this? No annoying wrinkles with age, no aching joints, no other diseases of old age, but eternal youth. Surely you have dreamed of this at one time or another. And you will see that although more active autophagy will not give you eternal youth, it will bring many other benefits if you support and further activate your body's own recycling system.

Autophagy is always active in cells in the normal state and runs in the background. However, in extreme situations, such as extreme cell damage, the cell can even initiate apoptosis or autophagosomal cell death. This means that it destroys itself and releases its resources to the surrounding cells. And what at first sounds like a pretty radical suicide program is actually an ingenious invention to ensure the survival of an entire organism. And this even benefits your immune system, because autophagy can also render pathogens such as viruses and bacteria harmless. In this way, cells can prevent viruses or bacteria that have entered the body from spreading further.

Unfortunately, however, autophagy also reaches its limits at some point and can no longer be used by the cells as they would like. With age, this process continues to decline and intracellular waste accumulates in the cells, which can no longer be recycled or can only be recycled slowly. If autophagy is inhibited, this leads to a cellular disaster, as many diseases are based on a reduced ability to autophagy, as this is how diseases such as diabetes, Alzheimer's or Parkinson's develop, and tumors and infectious diseases also have an easy time of it due to such a failure.

You can observe a cycle that you may be familiar with from your own home. As soon as you leave something lying around and put tidying and cleaning aside for a few days, a week later you find yourself in an apartment with stuff lying around in every corner, literally attracting the clutter. It's the same - or at least almost - in your cells. As soon as the first waste products accumulate that can no longer be broken down so quickly, the whole balance is thrown out of kilter and more and more waste accumulates in the cells and less and less can be broken down.

But you can count yourself lucky, because the research initiated by Yoshinori Ösumi has set a small cycle in motion that seems to be getting bigger and bigger: the search for ways to keep autophagy at a high level into old age. But before you rush to incorporate the possibilities already researched into your everyday life, full of zest for action and with the hope of prolonging the ageing process of your cells as much as possible, you will first learn more about the opportunity to make significant medical advances in the treatment of some diseases through this discovery in the next chapter.

# The great desire for healing

## DEMENTIA

Dementia is a disease that mainly affects older people and is characterized by forgetfulness, disorientation and difficulties in carrying out everyday tasks. After extensive research, scientists and doctors discovered that the disease is often caused by a lack of blood supply to the brain, which is caused by a circulatory disorder. This causes toxic proteins to stick together and lead to a narrowing of the blood vessels, as a result of which only some of the necessary nutrients reach the brain. However, together with research into auto-phagy, a way may also have been found to prevent the onset of dementia, as this recycling system can help the brain cells to cleanse themselves and destroy the toxic proteins. This prevents adhesions from forming in the first place and at least eliminates this cause of the disease. If you now boost the metabolism and autophagy of your cells, you can try to prevent dementia at an early stage.

Unfortunately, research in this area is still in its infancy and much is still unknown. However, scientists already agree that increased autophagy leads to a lower risk of developing dementia and can also be used as a therapy to slow down the progression of an existing disease.

## CANCER

Ever since the discovery and understanding of autophagy, cancer researchers have been certain that this cell property is of enormous importance when it comes to understanding tumors, because in order to cure cancer and tumors, it is first necessary to understand the process of development, which has long been misunderstood and is still not fully understood today. However, thanks to a laboratory experiment on mice whose cells were not capable of normal autophagy, doctors and scientists have already discovered that the lack of this ability actually leads to tumors occurring much more frequently and spontaneously.

But unfortunately, it's not quite that simple, because the problem is that dysfunctional autophagy can also contribute to cancer and help tumors grow. Dysfunctional autophagy means that the original function of cleaning cells and recycling waste products has been transformed. The affected cancer cells have taken over and give the lysosomes, which are responsible for autophagy, signals as to what they should do. This enables the cancer cells to produce products from the recycled substances that are useful to them and contribute to their proliferation. They can even fight against chemotherapy by breaking down the toxin introduced into the cells and thus producing new raw materials. All of this initially put the doctors in a very difficult position and they had to consider whether it made sense to promote autophagy or not.

Several studies then investigated how certain factors that stimulate autophagy affect cancer therapy or the course of the disease. One team of scientists found that substances contained in green tea have been shown to support autophagy, which leads to the death of tumor cells. Other researchers investigated the effectiveness of fasting on tumors and discovered that intermittent fasting can actually support chemotherapy and help to protect healthy cells, because by recycling waste products, healthy cells can rid themselves of their waste and gain new energy from it, which helps them to fight the tumor cells. In addition, the cells seem to tolerate chemotherapy better if patients stop eating a few hours before treatment and only eat again a few hours afterwards.

Autophagy can therefore not only help to prevent cancer, but also enable doctors to try out new treatment options that could perhaps also prevent the progression of an inoperable, aggressive tumor.

## AGEING

Surely none of you like to think about what you will look like in twenty or thirty years' time and what the ageing process will have done to you by then. This is understandable, because nobody likes to imagine how they will live with wrinkles, osteoarthritis and all kinds of other age-related illnesses. But once again, Japanese scientist Yoshinori Ōsumi has made it possible for you to escape this process a little by discovering autophagy. If you boost your autophagy metabolism, your cells can break down waste products more quickly and build new cell organelles from the recycled raw materials.

Now that scientists have discovered that the process of autophagy in cells decreases with age, you can conclude that you can delay your advancing age by additionally stimulating your cells to autophagy and ensuring that the waste products can continue to be broken down quickly. This means that you can not only prevent dementia or cancer, but also possibly extend your life by a few years.

## DIABETES

You will no doubt have heard about the many risks of diabetes and may also know that the pancreas does not produce enough insulin in this disease, resulting in an increased blood sugar level. Affected patients must therefore regularly measure their blood sugar levels and inject insulin if these levels are too high.

But to counteract type 2 diabetes in particular, autophagy is again of particular importance. Several studies have shown that autophagy protects the beta cells in the pancreas, which are responsible for insulin production. However, if autophagy is missing or no longer functions fully, these beta cells can be damaged and even stop producing insulin, thereby causing diabetes. By activating the cell metabolism, you can therefore both prevent diabetes and reverse type 2 diabetes itself, which would not be possible with diets alone, as is often recommended for diabetes.

## BRAIN

Autophagy, or rather the cessation of autophagy in the brain, has a somewhat surprising effect for scientists. Researchers from the Charité and the Leibniz-Forschungsinstitut für Molekulare Pharmakologie (FMP) have intensively studied autophagy and have come to the conclusion that in cells in which autophagy and thus the recycling process has been switched off by a genetic trick, there is not more unusable cell waste and proteins as expected, but an increased amount of endoplasmic reticulum. In addition to its function as a cell post, as you learned earlier, this is also responsible for calcium storage in the cells. More endoplasmic reticulum therefore leads to more calcium in the cells, which in turn leads to more neurotransmitters being released and the nerve cells being exposed to enormous over-excitation.

As autophagy plays a central role in the maintenance of cells and enables damaged, incorrect or foreign molecules to be broken down quickly, it is particularly important in the brain and for nerve cells. Unlike many other cells in the body, nerve cells cannot be completely renewed. They accompany you your whole life and if a nerve tears, it can only be repaired surgically. This makes it clear how important it is that nerve cells are preserved and not destroyed by incorrect or damaged organelles. Autophagy also prevents too many proteins from accumulating in the nerve cells and causing them to clump together, as is the case in neurodegenerative diseases. However, scientists now suspect that this protective effect may have completely different causes. At the FMP, they made an astonishing discovery through research on young and healthy mice:

In order to investigate the effect of autophagy, the scientists used a genetic trick to switch off autophagy in the nerve cells of the brain and then examined the protein content of these cells in detail. They noticed that proteins that they were actually sure were degraded by autophagy were not enriched in the cells, as would otherwise have been expected. Instead, however, they found something in the altered cells that was almost more surprising for them, because they found an increased amount of endoplasmic reticulum, which serves as a calcium store in all cells and regulates the transmission of excitation in nerve cells. However, it was precisely this important calcium store that was damaged in the altered cells and the researchers were able to prove that the calcium buffer function of the endoplasmic reticulum no longer worked properly. It was therefore no longer fully able to absorb free calcium and more free calcium remained in the nerve cell.

This in turn leads to hyperactivity of the cells, neurotransmitters are emitted continuously and they are actually permanently in an excited state. If autophagy had still functioned in these cells, the damaged endoplasmic reticulum would presumably have been renewed quickly and the cells would not have been damaged. However, in the event of such a functional failure, the endoplasmic reticulum that is no longer functioning properly remains and floods the cell with transmitters.

Until now, researchers have assumed that less autophagy also means that fewer transmitters are released due to the remaining cellular waste and damaged organelles and were therefore completely surprised by the results of the study. However, they now know that when there is a lack of autophagy, many more neuro-transmitters are present and the cells are therefore less malleable and also die from overexcitation. This could lead to an increased rate of cell death in affected areas of the brain and possibly also to a loss of function.

Scientists do not yet know much about the exact medical consequences and not much can be said about its involvement in diseases such as Alzheimer's or dementia. However, this new discovery has aroused the interest of researchers and doctors, who are certain that it will have a major impact on the treatment of degenerative diseases of the nervous system in the future.

## MUSCLE ATROPHY AND OSTEO-POROSIS

As a final point on the medical application of autophagy, you can read here about muscle atrophy and osteoporosis, which mainly occur in old age, but can also be triggered by a disease at a young age. However, researchers have now discovered that autophagy plays an important role in the progression and treatment of both diseases, as the body's own recycling process breaks down old or unusable products and can also decompose entire cells. New cells and cell components can then be produced from the resulting substances and a defective or infected cell cannot infect other cells.

As a result, more healthy muscle and bone mass is retained and osteoporosis and muscle atrophy can be delayed or even stopped altogether. However, it is also important to note that fasting and a calorie deficit, which leads to the activation of autophagy, can also result in the body lacking important nutrients such as proteins and calcium, which can exacerbate both problems. So when fasting and in a calorie deficit, make sure that you still provide your body with sufficient nutrients and do not completely eliminate important staple foods from your diet.

# Do it yourself

## HOW TO BOOST YOUR AUTO-PHAGY

But now, after all this exciting information, you come to the part where you can take action yourself. Do you want to support your cells, slow down your ageing process and do something for your health? Then you should now read carefully and remember the tips. And don't worry, it's not a great art to support your cells with autophagy and there are only a few points that speak in favor of giving it a try.

First, a brief recap of when autophagy is particularly active: Autophagic processes take place in all your cells at all times. In everyday life, their activity is rather low and negligible. The cells only do what is necessary and are more willing to absorb new resources from the environment.

However, certain factors can cause autophagy to stagnate. In addition to stress situations and irreparable cell damage that leads to cell death, this also includes a lack of nutrients. Particularly when amino acids are lacking, the cell begins to recycle more of its own waste products and to re-replenish unneeded organelles. However, if there are enough amino acids and other nutrients in the environment, the cell does not necessarily have to fall back on its own reserves and can also absorb new substances from the environment. And it is precisely at this point that you can become active yourself and support your cells in the autophagy of waste products. But first things first: you don't have to stop eating and starve yourself for days on end to achieve an effect. Read on and find out what small changes you can make today.

# THE FAST

You've probably heard of the infamous intermittent fasting and maybe you've even tried it yourself. However, if this is not the case, here is a brief explanation: Intermittent fasting, as the name suggests, involves fasting for a certain period of time and eating during the rest of the time. The best-known variant of this is probably the 16/8 method, where you fast for 16 hours a day and eat for eight hours. However, it is important to note that you should of course not eat for the whole eight hours, but spread your meals over this period. This means that you often automatically eat less and, in addition, the body has enough time in the following 16 hours to digest the food you have eaten sufficiently and absorb as many nutrients as possible.

In addition - as a bonus, so to speak - you can utilize your body's own waste products, because your body continues to need nutrients during the 16 hours of fasting, which it can then produce from its own unused products due to the lack of food and thus clean up the cells and utilize the waste.

If you go without food for a longer period of time, your insulin level remains at a constant low level and your body receives the signal that not enough energy has been taken in from outside. As a result, your body has to find other ways to get the energy it needs and begins to draw on its own energy reserves. Once the energy capacity of the fat cells is exhausted, your body looks for other sources of energy and begins to break down damaged and old cell structures, which brings you back to autophagy. Conversely, you can also say that frequent and excessive food intake inhibits this process and exactly the opposite happens, because your body absorbs so much energy that it doesn't really know what to do with it and therefore starts to build up fat reserves to prepare for worse times.

In summary, you can say that fasting and calorie reduction lead to a boost in your cell metabolism and the cells recycle cellular waste through autophagy. However, it is very important to remember that you should never fast too much or build up a huge calorie deficit, because the body is dependent on nutrients and energy from outside and the body cannot produce many products on its own. And you certainly don't want autophagy to turn your cells into little scavenger cells that greedily pounce on anything that gets in their way. Although stimulated autophagy supports your immune system, your immune system can also suffer greatly if you lack important vitamins and nutrients that you only get from food.

## SPORT

Another way to support your own recycling process in the cells is - how could it be otherwise - sport. If you look back a few millennia and think about how people lived in the Stone Age, you may notice that there were no gyms, sports clubs or the like and that sport was not necessarily a hobby, but rather the key to survival. If you couldn't run fast or put up enough of a fight against an attacker, you often lost out and lost the race against a sabre-toothed tiger or the fight for food, for example. For the body, sport and physical exertion were therefore much more of a stressful situation and the body sent signals to the cells to mobilize additional energy from the fat stores. As a result, the cells were also prompted to make greater use of their own waste products to obtain energy and nutrients.

Now, of course, you don't have to get into a similar situation and run away from a bear or tiger to achieve the same effect. As a study on mice showed, regular endurance exercise is enough to keep autophagy active. In this study, two groups of mice were fed a high-calorie, high-fat diet over a period of 13 weeks. The first group was allowed to remain lazy during this time and hardly moved at all, while the second group was regularly sent to a treadmill and made to exercise. After the period, the mice were examined and the researchers found that the mice from group one had gained a significant amount of weight and their blood values had also deteriorated. In group two, however, neither the weight nor the blood values changed negatively and autophagy was still at a high level. So the next time you are thinking about whether or not to go to the gym, just think about the fact that it not only releases happiness hormones and makes you feel fitter and better afterwards, but also that it allows you to run a little ahead of the ageing process and relieve your cells of all the ballast.

# SIRTFOOD

At this point, you are probably wondering what this is supposed to be and how it can be something that you actively incorporate into your everyday life. But behind this complex term is actually something very simple: sirtfoods are certain foods that can influence your metabolism and ageing process thanks to certain ingredients. But before you think that you have to change your entire diet and that sirtfood only consists of vegetables, here is a list of a few foods that count as sirtfood: In addition to some fruits and vegetables such as strawberries, chilies, onions, kale and blueberries, it also includes walnuts, buckwheat, chocolate with at least 80% cocoa content and even coffee and red wine. So you don't have to change your diet that much and can enjoy your next glass of red wine or piece of chocolate even more if you remember that you are actually doing something good for your body. But be careful! Too much red wine or chocolate can be a hindrance and reduce the activity of your cells.

These foods all contain sirtuin activators, which can boost your metabolism and, together with a calorie deficit, optimally help to activate your autophages. But again, remember that a lot does not always help a lot.

Don't overdo it and, above all, don't change too much at once. It will probably be a big change for your body and it should have the opportunity to get used to all the steps over time. This will help you achieve the best results and keep going for a long time. If you change everything from one day to the next, you will probably run out of energy after just a few weeks and stop trying. Use the weekly plan below as a guide and think about how you can incorporate it into your everyday life.

## FOOD

In addition to sirtfood, there are other foods that can support your metabolism and that you can easily incorporate into your daily routine, as nuts, mushrooms, apples, pears and black coffee also stimulate autophagy. However, when it comes to coffee, make sure that this only applies to black coffee. Milk contains protein and this nutrient inhibits the recycling activity of the cells.

Here are a few more foods in focus:

In the case of **coffee**, it is not necessarily the caffeine that stimulates autophagy in cells, but rather researchers suspect that it is certain antioxidants that create this benefit. It is not necessary to fast in order to obtain the activating effect, but you can also include a cup of coffee in your normal daily routine if you don't want to start fasting straight away. And before you can no longer sleep because of all the caffeine, you can also drink decaffeinated coffee, because as you have just read, the activating effect is not due to the caffeine, but rather to certain antioxidants.

**Olive oil** also has an activating effect on the metabolism and has a proven anti-cancer potential, which can presumably be attributed to its most important antioxidant, oleuropein. Surprising proof of this effect can be found in a village in southern Italy, where more than 300 people have lived to be over 100 years old and many older people showed hardly any signs of illnesses such as dementia or strokes. Incorporate a little more Mediterranean cuisine into your diet and support your cells with a dash of olive oil.

**Turmeric** has now also arrived in European cuisine and, in addition to its bright yellow color, turmeric also contains curcumin, an important substance for activating your cells. If you combine turmeric with black pepper when cooking, you get an even better effect and can even absorb 20 times as much curcumin. So what's wrong with a well-seasoned curry with a touch of black pepper and turmeric?

## SPERMIDINE

The last option for activating your autophages is the molecule spermidine, which was first discovered in human semen and years later was also found in all other body cells. This molecule has the property that it slows down the ageing process by increasing protein levels in the cells. However, the concentration decreases with increasing age, which is why additional spermidine should be made available to the body in old age through foods such as pulses, mushrooms, wheat germ or mature cheese. However, it is generally not recommended to resort to dietary supplements, but to obtain spermidine naturally.

A study that examined the concentration of spermidine in the blood, depending on age, found that the concentration, which is still at a high level at the age of 31 to 56, decreases significantly at the age of 60 to 80. In the study group aged 90 to 106, on the other hand, a high concentration was again determined, which even exceeded the value of the test subjects aged 31 to 51. The study therefore suggests that the few people who reach this age do so in connection with a high concentration of spermidine and a high level of autophagy activity.

# The way to the goal

On the last few pages, you have now learned a lot about how you can activate the recycling in your cells and are probably sitting on the edge of your chair full of energy and ready to get started. But first, take a step back and think about what you have learned and what you can and want to implement in your everyday life. It makes no sense to immediately fill your to-do list to the top and turn your life completely upside down. Instead, take things step by step and work through one item at a time.

# 1. PLANNING

Before you start with the exact implementation, make a plan and think about what you are already unconsciously doing in your everyday life that activates the autophagi. You are sure to find one or two foods in your kitchen and sport will certainly crop up in your everyday life at one time or another. Then realize once again what improvements such a change can bring you and how easily you can achieve them. Also consider whether you might want to tackle the "autophagy project" together with someone so that you can support each other and exercise or cook together. Such a change is always a little easier in pairs or in a small group and you can also share experiences with each other.

And finally, you should also consider whether you have any health problems that you should take into account in one respect or another. Not everyone's body is suitable for fasting, for example, and you should of course also take any intolerances into account.

Once you have clarified all these points, you can get started with the first part.

# 2 . START

You should use the first few weeks to get your bearings and find out what suits you and your everyday life. You won't run out of time and in a few weeks you can still really start to make an impact on your body. But it's better to take a little more time at the beginning to make a proper plan and check what's right for you. This will make things run much more smoothly in the active phase and you will know what you can fall back on.

In the beginning, you can continue to do the things that you have already unconsciously incorporated into your everyday life and plan them more consciously into your day. When you feel ready, you can also gradually approach intermittent fasting. If you already have experience in this area, you can of course start right away, but if you are new to all this, you should approach longer intervals step by step. We recommend starting with a 12/12 interval, which you can then gradually extend. As you also have to cope with your normal everyday life, you should not expose your body to too many new and strenuous situations at once. You have enough time and it's not a problem if you don't make the progress you want to for a few weeks. In the end, everything always turns out differently than expected.

In the first few weeks, it is therefore a good idea to make a few notes about what you have changed and how it has affected your day and how you feel. Did the change feel good or bad? Did you feel a change? Does it work even in times when you are more stressed? The most important thing in this phase is not to get overconfident, but to listen to your body, because it will definitely tell you how it feels. If you notice that something is not going well for you, don't grit your teeth and fight through it, but change your plan a little and continue on a new path. If you have had little to do with the points for activating autophagy before, it can also be good if you choose a specific area to start with and begin with either fasting, calorie deficit, exercise or a change in diet. Of course, all points belong together, but just as too many cooks spoil the broth, you will not achieve good long-term results if you do everything at once.

# 3. DO NOT GIVE UP

As with all things, there will be moments when you want to give up and abandon the whole project. It is precisely in these phases that you should remind yourself exactly why you are doing the whole thing. As a little help, you can also write down the points and hang them up somewhere in your home where you can read them again and again. And don't forget that everyone has a bad day and things don't go as planned. If you have such a day, it is only important that you get back into a routine over the next few days. It's not a problem if you skip exercise, the fast doesn't work the way you want it to or you have a "cheat day", it's even good if you reward yourself with a good meal or don't follow the plan completely, as this will make it more fun again afterwards and make it easier for you to stick to it.

The only rule is not to throw your autophagy activation plan overboard and forget everything you have learned. The better you stick to the plan, the easier it is for the cells to maintain a consistently high level of metabolic activity. However, if you keep switching back and forth and don't have the right structure in everything, your cells will also be a bit overwhelmed and you won't achieve the desired result. So remember that cheat days are not a problem and that you can sometimes neglect your plan. It's normal if you lose interest from time to time and need a bit of variety, but always come back to your actual goal and help your cells to free themselves from all the garbage.

# 4. IMPATIENCE

With all the change you have now undergone, you are probably expecting or hoping to feel a significant change soon. However, you need to remind yourself once again what your goals are. You want to counteract your ageing process by ridding your cells of useless products and you also want to support your immune system and prevent diseases in old age.

These are all points that you only become aware of over time or not at all. After all, you don't know what things would have been like without your new lifestyle. Perhaps you would have been ill much more often in recent months, perhaps you would be diagnosed with dementia in old age or die a few years earlier. Unfortunately, you have no way of knowing. Perhaps you would have been just as well off with your old lifestyle as you are now. But if you are one of the few people who doesn't fall ill during the cold season, or if you are still much fitter at 60 than your friends and colleagues of the same age, then you can be sure that this change has contributed to this. And before you are disappointed that you don't see any direct effect, read on.

Regular exercise will generally make you feel better, more relaxed and more productive. Sport also builds muscle, burns fat, releases happiness hormones and prevents depression. You can cope better with stressful phases at work or in everyday life and are better able to deal with problems. You will also get better at sport every time you exercise and will be able to achieve more and more. Isn't it great when you keep improving at jogging, for example, and can eventually run distances you never even dreamed of a year ago?

If you also build a calorie deficit into your plan, i.e. you consume more calories than you take in, you will shed excess pounds and your body will be generally healthier. But again, make sure you eat the right amount and don't overdo it! Losing weight too quickly is not healthy and you should not lose too much weight. If you are already at a healthy weight that you feel comfortable with, then stick to it and cross this item off your list. The body also needs a lot of energy and nutrients to build muscle, which you would deprive it of by not eating enough. If your body doesn't get these nutrients from outside, it will start to break down underused muscles itself, which is the opposite of what you want to achieve. So the important thing to remember is: a calorie deficit is fine if it doesn't harm your health or your body and you don't give up too much at once!

Another point that you will quickly notice is that you are more balanced and lead a generally happier life. You won't be so easily upset and because your body will feel better, you and your mind will also feel better. It's amazing what positive effects changing so few things can have, isn't it?

## 5. CAUTION

In the previous text, you have already repeatedly come across small warnings, which are briefly summarized below.

**Change:** It's great if you want to change something in your life and do more for your health, but remember that your body needs time and will only get used to everything gradually. It's better to go step by step and not do everything at once. This way you can also track how your body reacts to the individual steps and whether you tolerate them well or not.

**Fasting:** Before you start, you should definitely consider to what extent this is possible with your everyday life and work. If you have a physically demanding job and need a lot of energy from an early age, the 16/8 method may not be right for you. To start with, you can also choose individual days on which you try out different methods and then see which one works best for you.

**Calorie deficit: It is** particularly important here that you do not overdo it. Your body needs a lot of energy throughout the day just to function normally and if you also do more sport, your calorie requirement will increase even further. So before you start going without, you should be clear about how much energy you need per day. If you are already at a healthy weight, do not reduce it any further, but rather try to build up more muscle. The body also needs a lot of energy and important nutrients such as protein, which it can absorb through food. If you are unsure, ask your family doctor what his opinion is and what he would recommend.

**Impatience:** Of course you want to be rewarded as soon as possible for your change and your renunciation, but don't be too impatient, instead pay attention to the small positive changes. Unfortunately, many successes will not be immediately visible to you and will happen rather unconsciously, but rest assured: your decision was the right one and you are doing something good for your body and your health and even

preventing illnesses in old age. Give your body time -
after all, it takes several years for a seed to become a
fruit-bearing tree.

50

# 6. WHAT ARE YOU STILL WAITING FOR?

Now that you have learned so much and know how you can support your cells to keep the recycling process going for longer, nothing stands in your way of better health and possibly a longer life. You have all the information you need and just need to put it into practice. Get started right away and look for a few suitable recipes, plan your next exercise session or find a club near you where you can get active together in a group from time to time.

You will soon realize that this change is not such a big change and you will automatically incorporate it into your day. After a few months, you may not even be able to imagine what it was like before, and you'll be glad you discovered this book and didn't stop reading on the first page when it started talking about biology, school and cells. Do something for your health and that of others and shine with your knowledge at the next family celebration or get-together with friends and encourage those around you to join the autophagy club.

# Autophagy vs. pandemic

Finally, in the last chapter, you can learn more about the benefits of more active cell autophagy against the coronavirus, because even in the current situation, in which the world is in the middle of a pandemic, the researched importance of coronaviruses on autophagy in cells opens up a new possibility for therapy. In the search for possible drugs to combat the severe symptoms of an infection, researchers from Berlin and Bonn worked together to investigate the effect that virus cells have on the body's cells and how they reprogram the cells' metabolism to help them spread further in the body. Through this research, they discovered that SARS-CoV-2 can slow down or even completely disrupt the recycling mechanism of cells by interfering with autophagy. However, as you already know, autophagy is important for cells to break down waste products and cellular invaders and produce new substances.

In one study, scientists then made the decisive discovery that the virus makes use of the organisms and cell structures and even manipulates the metabolism by simulating to the cell that sufficient food is available. This means that it is not necessary for the cell to start the process of autophagy and thus recycle new usable substances from its own products. The coronaviruses are thus able to avoid autophagic degradation and can survive longer in the host.

Thanks to these research findings, doctors and scientists may have found a new starting point for a therapy. Following the discoveries they made about the connection between coronaviruses and autophagy, they have now investigated a number of active substances that have been proven to stimulate autophagy, hoping for a positive effect and containment of the virus.

And they actually found four substances that proved to be effective against the coronavirus, all of which are already on the market and are used elsewhere in medicine. In addition to spermine and spermidine, which you have already seen, a cancer drug and even the tapeworm drug niclosamide also showed a very effective effect. The tapeworm drug actually had the greatest effect and the production of new coronaviruses in cells was reduced by more than 99%. This discovery is a great success for the doctors, as niclosamide is already approved and the side effects and possible long-term consequences have already been intensively investigated and the tolerable dosage is also known, this drug can soon also be prescribed against coronaviruses and help to contain or even prevent a severe course of the disease.

As part of a clinical study, scientists in Berlin are now investigating the extent to which niclosamide achieves positive effects in patients. So far, the efficacy has only been proven in the laboratory and now the aim is to find enough volunteers to hopefully demonstrate a positive effect in patients. A phase 2 study called NICCAM is currently being initiated to investigate how well or whether niclosamide, when given together with the drug Camostat, is effective against coronaviruses and - at least as importantly - whether patients tolerate the drug well. Unfortunately, it will be some time before the results of the study are evaluated and the drugs can be used in this combination against corona. But fortunately, other drugs have also shown an effect.

In the laboratory, it was shown that when spermidine was administered, the cells produced 85% fewer virus particles and when spermine was administered, the figure was even higher at 90%. This result is wonderful, because spermine and spermidine are endogenous substances that the cells can produce themselves and that can also be supplied via certain foods. This therefore promises a high level of tolerability and the approval of such drugs should also be much faster. However, there is a problem here, because in the laboratory the researchers used both substances in a pure form, which as such is not suitable for ingestion as medication. However, spermidine in particular was only effective at a very high concentration, which cannot be achieved through a special diet alone. There are therefore still many unanswered questions regarding these active substances and scientists still have a long way to go before spermine and spermidine can actually be used as antidotes.

The last active ingredient mentioned, a cancer drug, has so far only been tested in the laboratory for both its anti-cancer and anti-corona effects. Approval in the near future can therefore be ruled out from the outset. However, in a study at the Charité hospital in Berlin, doctors have already been able to prove that the cancer drug MK-2206 reduces virus production by around 90% and is therefore also effective against this virus. However, it is still necessary to test what possible side effects the drug has on patients and what effect can be achieved at what dose. So there is a light at the end of the tunnel, but it will still be a long and arduous journey to get there.

# To the point

You have now learned a lot of new things and you may need to read some of them again. You have learned how cells are structured and which components are crucial for cell survival. You also now know what medical possibilities have arisen from research into autophagy and that the Japanese scientist Yoshinori Ösumi was quite rightly awarded the Nobel Prize for his research. And best of all, you have even learned how to support your own cells and immune system and plan the path to a happier and healthier life. You can now start to prevent disease as you age and ensure that you live a longer and more active life. And it's all because the cells like to have order and be self-sufficient, because they prefer to get rid of their waste right away and not waste anything in the process. This little process of autophagy, which probably seemed very abstract to you at first and by no means so crucial for your health, is a true masterpiece and thanks to this discovery, medicine will change significantly in the coming years and decades.

And perhaps the global economy will also discover a similar recycling system for itself and start taking the absolutely necessary measures for a better climate. If not only the smallest subunits of the human being - the cells - were so careful not to waste energy and raw materials and to correct errors as early as possible so that no more damage is done, but also the entire human organism, then there would probably be no shortage of raw materials, mountains of waste that are getting bigger and bigger, or disposable plastic bags, shrink-wrapped fruit and vegetables and much more. Humanity is therefore facing a major turning point not only in the field of medicine and treatment, but hopefully soon also in the use of raw materials and the sustainable consumption of resources.

Perhaps you would also like to cleanse your body and cells as well as your environment and make it more sustainable. Not only does it only take a few small changes to your cells to achieve a significant effect, but it is also possible to achieve sustainability in everyday life. As with your cells, it is also important that many individual units work together.

It is no good if only one cell becomes more active, it must also encourage more and more cells in its environment to become more active and follow its example. You too can start by taking your own bags to the shops, buying fruit and vegetables openly, cycling more and much more, and encouraging your friends and family to join in. This will motivate more and more people and together you will achieve a great effect, even though each individual has only made a small change. Why not make a little game out of it with your family or circle of friends? Which of you manages to leave the car at home the most? Who buys the least packaged items when shopping? Who uses packaging - only if possible, of course - more than once? There are so many ideas and it's much more fun together than alone. Don't just take something from this book for yourself and your health, but also think about your environment and the generations that will come after you!